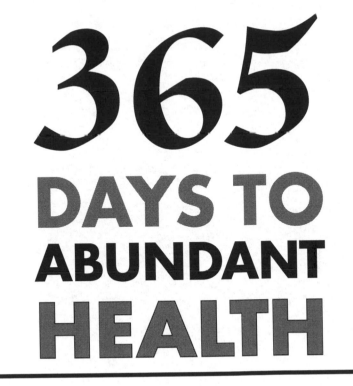

365

DAYS TO
ABUNDANT
HEALTH

The Little Steps That Help You Thrive

KIM M. WHITE

BALBOA
PRESS

A DIVISION OF HAY HOUSE

Balboa Press books may be ordered through booksellers or by contacting:

Balboa Press
A Division of Hay House
1663 Liberty Drive
Bloomington, IN 47403
www.balboapress.com
1 (877) 407-4847

Because of the dynamic nature of the Internet, any web addresses or links contained in this book may have changed since publication and may no longer be valid. The views expressed in this work are solely those of the author and do not necessarily reflect the views of the publisher, and the publisher hereby disclaims any responsibility for them.

The author of this book does not dispense medical advice or prescribe the use of any technique as a form of treatment for physical, emotional, or medical problems without the advice of a physician, either directly or indirectly. The intent of the author is only to offer information of a general nature to help you in your quest for emotional and spiritual well-being. In the event you use any of the information in this book for yourself, which is your constitutional right, the author and the publisher assume no responsibility for your actions.

Any people depicted in stock imagery provided by Thinkstock are models, and such images are being used for illustrative purposes only.
Certain stock imagery © Thinkstock.

Print information available on the last page.

ISBN: 978-1-5043-3359-7 (sc)
ISBN: 978-1-5043-3361-0 (hc)
ISBN: 978-1-5043-3360-3 (e)

Library of Congress Control Number: 2015908705

Balboa Press rev. date: 06/18/2015

Contents

Foreword

Have you ever played this game? You've decided to see what message the universe might have for you, so you pick up a book and open it at random to see the first thing that catches your eye. How many times did we just happened to find the very statement that could change our day or perhaps even our life? This is what I love about Kim's wonderful book. There's something in it for everyone! Who of us wouldn't like to improve our heath, fitness and well being? Imagine just how wonderful you'll feel knowing you now have the tools for maintaining youthfulness at any age?

These short little tips are truly gems. Here's another way you can go through this book. If you like, just take one insight each day and apply the suggestion. I promise, you'll find this practice transforming. All it takes is just one idea to transform your life. Thankfully, Kim has given you one for each day of the year. I hope you'll be as excited as I've been to read and apply the tips in this book!

Peter Ragnar, The Longevity Sage

Acknowledgments

I would like to first thank God (aka. Source, Universal Intelligence, or whatever you wish to call it) for giving me the strength to do everything. Also, to my parents, Hal and Pauline who have always been a source of love and support. To my aunt, Jan Toom who encourages me in writing and any of my quests.

My gratitude goes out to the Global Information Network (G.I.N.) whose system gave me the self-esteem and persistence to know that I can be, do and have anything and everything I want in life. To Kevin Trudeau who started the club and the AXS Consulting, LLC who has kept the club moving forward with integrity. To Troy McClain for his support, encouragement and definition of luck.

Thanks go out to my friends who screened the book: Nancy Utovac, Lucrecia Jacobson and Lori Johnson. My appreciation goes out to all of my friends who have been there for me during this endeavor: from the Cabrillo Beach Polar Bear club, San Pedro Elk's Lodge No. 966, Mission Eben-Ezer Family Church; G.I.N. Local Chapter - Los Angeles and all of those I've known on this joyous journey. Special thanks go to those who always inspire me and support me: Beth Sanden, Ellen Morgan, Becca Morgan, all my CAF friends, and Brenda Swanney.

Thanks go to Peter Ragnar for writing the foreward to this book. He is such a wise soul and has such a love for living a truly happy, healthy and long life.

Introduction

Everybody wants to improve their health, but not many know how.

This book has practical tips that any person can do so they can do just that.

Every day, you can make a change in what you eat, how you move or what you think that will improve your health and your life. This book is set up to try one each day, lasting an entire year. Once your year is complete, you can repeat it or gift it to a friend.

My secret wish and desire is that you would not try this idea for one day but try the idea and keep it and add on the next idea the next day and add it on until all of these become a part of your life.

Some of the ideas may not resonate with you and that's okay. If you are able, try it anyways or try something similar. You can make adaptations to some of the ideas in this book.

One definition of insanity is doing the same thing over and over expecting different results. - Chinese Proverb

You have a choice. You can try to do one of these changes every single day of the year, which is how this book was meant to be read. The other option is to make one of these changes per week and then the book will last a lot longer. It may be easier, but you won't see as great of changes in your body. It's your choice how often you wish to add another one in to your daily regimen, but do it and do it now!

I have spent years exercising and trying to lose weight. I have spent money on pills, fad diets and exercised like a professional. I have been frustrated to my wits end. I understand how you feel. I felt the same way. Let me explain what I've found.

I have seen clients do the exercise, but refuse to change their diet. Most programs focus upon the changes you make to your body which happen in two different ways, though exercise and changing your diet. But there is another aspect: how you think and feel about the changes you are making. You must also address your thoughts as well as diet and exercise. I'm not saying that this will be easy. Nothing of great value is easy to do, but know that you are worth it!

Your body can see change in two different forms of exercise, through strength training and through cardiovascular exercise. There are many different types of cardiovascular exercise. There are the commonly known running, cycling, swimming, aerobic classes, martial arts and yoga classes. Yet, there are many more. Feel free to check out the internet to find all of the different types of exercise you can try. You can also try the latest type of class and see if you like it. If one class doesn't appeal to you, that is okay. I used to love rollerskating or ice skating. Sometimes I still go and do those things. Just know that you need to find exercise that you enjoy so that you will keep doing it. If what you are doing is no longer fun, try something else. There is no rule that you must stay with the same thing all of your life. It is better for your body to change your form of exercise every four to six weeks so that your body doesn't get bored or complacent. You will see greater changes in your body when you change what you do with it.

Strength training is another component of exercise to body change. It makes you stronger and leaner. You could go to a gym or try a program at home. There are numerous videos out to help you. It is better if you seek help from a professional Personal Trainer to make sure that you have proper form. Doing the exercises correctly will keep you from injury. You may wish to see a trainer on a regular basis for motivation and to make sure you are doing the exercises correctly. If you have good discipline, the trainer could be seen occasionally, like a tune up for your car.

Another component of your body's fitness is stretching. You need to keep your body limber. Stretching after exercise is a good way to loosen the muscles after a walk or any workout. Taking a yoga or Pilates class can help also. There are videos for both of these. There are other tools such as a Foam Roller and other tools to help you stay flexible. Again, check the internet to see what is available. I have found that most people will actually do what is on the videos if they like it. Feel free to rent videos before you buy so that you know if you like the instructor and feel like you will do the workout.

Now, let's talk about food. I'm not trying to get anyone to go "on a diet." Those usually don't work for a long time. I'm suggesting that if you change your dietary habits and eat a healthier diet, you will be making a lifestyle change. Your diet makes up about 80% of the changes you can make to your body.

It is important to eat a healthy diet, but there is so much conflicting information out there. There are three different kinds of Macronutrients: proteins, carbohydrates and fats. We need portions of each every day. What percentage we need of each is always under scrutiny. I suggest discussing this with your doctor or a nutritionist. I have found that having under 20% of fat, works best for me. The proteins and carbohydrates change depending upon how much exercise I am performing. My body prefers that I get most of my carbohydrates from fruits and vegetables. In appendix A and B, I have included the most common and some different fruits and vegetables. This list is not all inclusive, as there are many more fruits and vegetables from different areas of the world. I would suggest that you could try different ones from the list. Consider experimenting with seasonings and toppings to change the flavors until you find ones that you like.

Another key to this process is Love. You have to love yourself and know that you are worth the effort to become healthier. It is not selfish to improve yourself and your health. It is essential! It is essential to your health and without your health, you can not help someone else to the best of your ability. This idea is exemplified by the emergency procedures that are instructed by flight attendants: you must put your oxygen mask on yourself before putting one on your child or someone else.

So, love yourself first. Take care of your health first. Then, you can better take care of others. If you 'play full on' and do the items suggested in this book, you will see great changes in your life. Then others may want to know what you did and how you did it. You could give them a copy of this book or just recommend it to them.

In working on your mind, work on getting your mind to think more positively. There are many ways that you can do this: reading books that enrich your life; listening to positive audios (CD's or mp3's); going to seminars in your area with motivational speakers; or simply just repeating affirmations such as, "every day in every way, I'm getting better and better." There are positive statements sprinkled throughout this book which you can use, or you could search the internet for an affirmation that resonates with your heart. I suggest that you repeat it three times a day for at least 21 days.

One way to stay motivated is to join a group or create one where there are other people on a similar journey. There are organized groups that have programs attached to them. You could start a group in your neighborhood, among your friends, at your church or synagog, or within a larger club. When you hang around other people with the same goals, you can motivate each other and you can recognize when fellow members reach a big goal or even a smaller intermediary goal, such as doing the items on the list, staying positive or losing a couple pounds.

There is no quick cure. There is no magic pill. If you want to lose weight and get fit, you have to make changes in your life. This is easier said than done.

What I propose is a step-by-step process to improve your health by making small, positive changes in your life. Do it in your own time. Let the only person who pushes you be you. Unless you are told by your medical doctor that you must do a lot immediately, I suggest making one change every day.

Before beginning any exercise program, consult your doctor. If you are taking any medication, let your doctor know about the changes you are about to undertake. Some medications may react to healthy foods. I believe it is better to be safe than sorry.

As I mentioned before your diet is a big portion of weight gain or loss and body fat percentage (as much as 80%.) I prefer using body fat percentage (%) over Body Mass Index (BMI.) BMI measures height to weight ratio which is fine for the regular person. For those who already exercise or for athletes, BMI may be inaccurate. For example, through measuring body fat percentage hydrostatically (water weighing,) I had 21.3 % body fat which is considered lean. But when measuring my BMI, the number was 31 which is considered Obese. It was a terrible blow to the self esteem which made me depressed. Consider the best test for you based upon accuracy and cost.

Body fat percentage can be calculated at a gym with calipers or it can be calculated at home with a scale that has Bio-electrical impedance which is safe. The most accurate, but also most expensive way to measure body fat is through Hydrostatic weighing where you are in a dunked in a water tub just after exhaling and being weighed. It can be scary if you fear water or do not like exhaling and holding your breath.

Whatever method you choose, do not get the measurement to judge yourself harshly. Do it to get a base line or start point. Then, after a year when you finish this book, you can do another test to see just how far you've come.

With that being said, let us start your journey to abundant health. Know that there may be hiccups or challenges along the way, but know that you can always pick up where you left off and begin again.

I have designed this book so that you can choose to tear out a page each week. One side of the paper will have an affirmation, mantra or quotation that can be your focus for the week. The other side will have seven changes you can make that week.

There is one last thing that I want you to know before you begin this journey: You are perfect where you are right now, whatever your body looks like, and however you feel. This life is a learning experience and you are where you need to be right now. Just work on feeling a little bit better and doing a little bit better for yourself.

Take control of your life. Make the changes. Enjoy the process!

Let's start your journey...

"Write it on your heart that every day is the best day in the year."[i]

- Ralph Waldo Emerson

1. Although it's great to have role models on your path to health, remember that they may have started from a different place. If you can find someone who has been where you are, see if you can find a Biography or Auto-biography about them. Start reading the book. Start today & just work on improving a little bit at a time.

2. Drink more water (add one 8 oz. glass weekly to your daily intake until you are up to 8 - 12 glasses per day) – more when you exercise!

3. Eat one more piece of fruit today.

4. Eat one more vegetable today.

5. Move for 5 minutes more today than yesterday.

6. Cut down on sugary products.

7. Read labels on your food.

"Always bear in mind that your resolution to succeed is more important than any one thing."[ii]

Abraham Lincoln

8. Cut down on salt today.

9. Men: if your lower back is achey or keeps going out, consider moving your wallet out of your back pocket while sitting. Maybe you can use the inside pocket of your jacket.

10. Ask yourself why you want to change. Is it for you or someone else?

11. Drink one less sugary drink today.

12. Keep a food diary (including how you FEEL when you put something in your mouth.)

13. If you exercise for a long period of time (over 1 hour,) make sure that you have ample fuel. Fuel = water, electrolyte beverage & food (if hot weather, stick to beverages; if colder, add more solid fuel (energy bars or PB&J sandwiches.))

14. Feeling hungry? Drink a full 8oz. glass of water and wait 15 minutes to see if you still are.

"Great things are
done by a series
of small things
brought together."[iii]

Vincent Van Gogh

15. Eat a big salad first with your meal.

16. While dining out, ask the server to put half of your meal in a to go box before it is served.

17. Are you at Happy Hour & can't find anything healthy? Look at the ingredients on the menu & ask if they can make a salad from them with protein on it.

18. Try a piece of fruit and a small handful of nuts for a snack between meals.

19. Drink one LESS glass of soda pop today.

20. Decrease the amounts of grains in your diet today.

21. A good nights sleep is key...have a set routine you do before going to bed each night & it will signal your brain to comply.

"We change when the pain to change is less than the pain to remain as we are."[iv]

Ed Foreman, U.S. Congressman (Ret.) Texas & New Mexico, Author, Speaker, Entrepreneur

22. Put on your favorite song and dance.

23. Walk around the block (if it's not safe to be outside, walk 5 – 10 minutes inside your home.)

24. When walking, swing your arms.

25. Take the dog for a walk (or a neighbor's dog.)

26. Position yourself 2 inches forward on your chair & use your abdominal muscles to keep your back straight instead of the chair back. (Start with 10-15 minutes a day and work your way up to more time each day.)

27. Wake up 15 minutes earlier (and exercise.)

28. Do not compare yourself with someone else...only track your progress. Each person has a different body with different levels of hormones & toxins in it. Just try to be a little bit better today than you were yesterday.

"Life is not merely being alive, but being well."[v]

Marcus Valerius Martialis

29. Pull your belly button toward your spine (using only the tummy muscles.)

30. Don't add salt at the table.

31. Going out with friends and plan on drinking? Drink one glass of water between each alcoholic beverage.

32. Coming back after an injury has healed? Start out easy & work your way up slowly. You will get your fitness levels back. Hint: watch the calories you take in. Don't eat as much if you are not burning the calories.

33. Write down 5 things you are grateful for before bed.

34. Go outside and actually smell the roses (or another flower.)

35. If you smoke, smoke one less today.

"The happiness of your life depends upon the quality of your thoughts."[vi]

Marcus Aurelius

36. Put the remote on a table across the room from your chair so you have to get up and go get it to change the channel or volume.

37. Make healthier choices when ordering out (i.e. salad with chicken.)

38. Breathe in...deep...fill up the lungs, starting with the belly, expand the ribs, then the shoulders come up...then exhale. Repeat at least 3-10 times.

39. If you have a realistic goal of someone's body you'd like to look like, get their picture, cut & paste your head on it & put it on your dream board.

40. Park at the farthest spot in the parking lot.

41. If you'd like to try a healthy dessert, consider cinnamon on a baked apple or sweet potato.

42. Choose Organic over traditional (hint: in season is cheaper.)

"In health there is freedom. Health is the first of all liberties."[vii]

Henri Frederic Amiel

43. Company or club potluck? Bring something healthy & take bigger portions of healthy stuff. Take small tablespoon size tastes of not-so-healthy foods.

44. Bring workout clothes to work (so you are ready at the end of the day.)

45. Have a protein snack after your workout to rebuild the body.

46. How do Supermodels stay in their skinny jeans? When the jeans get snug, they eat a little bit less.

47. It's okay to leave something on your plate (or Fedex the leftovers to China.)

48. There are a few reasons to drink sparkling water at the holiday parties: no DUI, not making a fool of yourself, watching others acting stupid & no liquid calories.

49. Keep chemicals like Magnesium Stearate, Stearic Acid and Talc OUT of your supplements and products.

"Your aim should be to do what you can with what you have."[viii]

Theodore Roosevelt

50. Need a fitness goal? Sign up for a race and train for it.

51. Read labels on the hair and body products that you use. (Chemicals to avoid: see appendix D.)

52. Make your goals easy to attain so that you set yourself up for success!

53. Challenge yourself and see how many days you can go without your favorite guilty pleasure food. If it's not one month, try one week; if it's not one week, try one day; if not one day, try one hour...then try to increase it each try.

54. If you falter one day, just pick up where you left off. It's just one day.

55. Try the 80/20 Rule – eat healthy 80% of the time and allow yourself not so good foods 20% of the time.

56. Take a Multi-Vitamin (especially if you are on a diet.)

"Knowing is not enough, we must apply. Willingness is not enough, we must do."[ix]

Johann von Goethe

57. When moving heavier objects at home, protect your back by using your legs more. Make frequent stops to rest. You may be able to get 2 sets of 10 squats in that way. Stretch afterwards.

58. Do tricep dips at your desk.

59. Flying somewhere, do heel pumps: putting a little weight on your legs (like leaning forward) raise your heals 10 times. Repeat every couple hours on longer flights to avoid blood clots. Or you can walk to the restroom and back.

60. If your desk is against a wall, do push-ups with your hands on your desk.

61. Keep your knees directly above your heels when doing lunges.

62. Use 16 ounce cans of food to do bicep curls at home.

63. Use those 16 oz. cans to work your shoulders by pressing them over your head.

"The rung of a ladder was never meant to rest upon, but only to hold a man's foot long enough to enable him to put the other somewhat higher."[x]

Thomas Huxley

64. Going to a wedding or formal party? Consider drinking soda water with lime. It is bubbly so that you can toast with the champagne drinkers.

65. Eat your salad last, so it can move other food through your digestive tract.

66. If you want to strengthen your abs, try a plank. Start on your hands and knees keeping your body straight between your head & knees. Work your way up to a straight plank with hands & feet. Progress to side planks.

67. Find a work-out buddy (human or canine.)

68. Pull your belly button into your spine while doing all abdominal exercises.

69. Pull in your belly button while driving when you see a red light or stop sign.

70. In the evening, jog in place in front of the television.

"You can't hate yourself happy. You can't criticize yourself thin. You can't shame yourself wealthy.

Real change begins with self love and self care."[xi]

Jessica Ortner

71. When clipping coupons, clip for healthy snacks and avoid junk food coupons.

72. When in the market, mainly shop around the edges of the store.

73. Take a chance and try something new...a ballroom or salsa dance class!

74. Stressed at the end of the night? Don't reach for food, reach for a pen & a cup of tea. Drink the tea while writing down your stresses. Then you won't stay awake thinking about them because you know you can return to your writings.

75. When walking, do speed-play – at every other mailbox, push it a little faster to the next one, then back off and repeat.

76. Make playlists of music for specific workouts.

77. Bring one resistance band on vacation and you can keep your strength training up.

"We are what we repeatedly do. Excellence then, is not an act, but a habit."[xii]

Aristotle

78. Write your own affirmation & carry it on an index card & read it aloud 4 times a day.

79. Watch a silly comedy that you love and laugh, let loose.

80. While you are driving, listen to upbeat music and squeeze your buns to the beat…together, right bun only, left bun only.

81. Crazy hours at work? Don't know when you'll get a chance to eat? Bring many healthy, energizing snacks with you & munch at each break.

82. Buy a rebounder/mini-trampoline and bounce to your favorite music.

83. Allow yourself a small amount of your favorite sinful delight (like one Hershey's Kiss.)

84. Eat as much protein as the size of palm of your hand (without the fingers.)

"To keep the body in good health is a duty, otherwise we shall not be able to keep our mind strong and clear."[xiii]

Buddha

85. When cooking, exchange butter for Extra Virgin Olive Oil.

86. Laugh.

87. Home late from work & feel HUNGRY? Reach for something healthy first & a big glass of water, then wait 30 min & decide if you need more.

88. Burn a few extra calories by using chop sticks while eating.

89. Exchange your salad plate and your large dinner plate. Put salad on the dinner plate and your main dish on the salad plate.

90. If you are taking care of a child, parent or loved one, find workouts you can do at home: treadmill or walk/pace around the house; get a stationary bike or put yours on a trainer (stationary device for your bike); dance to music; exercise with bands or home weight lifting.

91. At your desk or in your car, put a sticky note in a prominent place to remind you to straighten your posture. Roll your shoulders back & down, then push your chin straight back like a turtle.

"There is no failure except in no longer trying."[xiv]

Elbert Hubbard

92. Set an appointment with yourself to workout.

93. Make a healthy birthday goal – run one mile (or lap) for every year or a mile per year on the bike or a lap in the pool per year or 1 minute of dancing per year of life.

94. Use the app on your phone to remind you to get up and move (even at work.)

95. Eat a variety of vegetables & fruits daily.

96. Neck feeling tight? Take time to stretch it: lean to the left & right, front, around to the left and right (hold for 30 seconds each way.)

97. Eating out with family at a place with a less-than-healthy menu? Choose the healthiest item on the menu & have steamed veggies for the side.

98. When you stretch, don't bounce or force it, stretch to stretch, not to pain.

"Know ye not that ye are the temple of God, and that the Spirit of God dwelleth in you?"[xv]

1 Corinthians 3:16 (KJV)

99. Don't eat food with added sugar. If you must have sugar, eat it specifically because you want it (like a SMALL candy bar.)

100. If you work with your hands, take a break occasionally & stretch your hands: putting your palms together and bending the fingers back, maybe doing a little hand massage. This will help your hands feel invigorated.

101. Going up the escalator & no one ahead of you? Treat the escalator like a stair case & get up there faster for some exercise.

102. Married? Sex burns calories. Hint: the person on top burns more calories.

103. Smile! People will wonder what you're thinking about.

104. Worked out hard all week? Take a rest day, eat some protein but not too many calories... Let your muscles heal.

105. Traveling? Use the airports gym or (on the cheap) just walk up & down the concourse while awaiting your flight or baggage.

"He who has health, has hope. And he who has hope, has everything."[xvi]

Thomas Carlyle

106. After a meal, take a walk. This will help your food digest better than sitting still.

107. Eat breakfast every day (even if it's only some yogurt.)

108. A glass of wine is 90 calories…burn that by walking or running a mile.

109. Inner thighs rub together? Use Sport Slick, BodyGlide, Tri-Slide Silicone Gel, Spanx, or wear long shorts to avoid chafing.

110. Do a "sit-to-stand" exercise at your desk by going from a seated position and standing up. Come back slowly. Repeat ten times.

111. If you have allergies, try LOCAL organic honey. The bees are getting pollen from local flowers and the honey should help your immunity.

112. Apple Cider Vinegar in water daily has been known to help with allergies and weight loss.

"Our greatest glory is not in never falling, but in getting up every time we do."[xvii]

Confucius

113. Consider doing a cleanse or detox once a quarter or you can just try one and see how you feel.

114. Hot summer day? Go for a swim.

115. Want something sweet, try an herbal tea with Cinnamon or add Stevia leaf.

116. Flying? Make sure you drink a little extra water since the air system dries out the air in the plane.

117. Feel like you've taken too much time off your workouts? Start now. Even a 5 minute walk will help. Work up to three 10 minute walks per day.

118. At a conference? Do a walking meeting. You can discuss business while moving. Exercise and work!

119. Bored with your workout? Try something different like martial arts or the newest style class at the gym.

"One can have no greater or smaller mastery than mastery of one's self."[xviii]

Leonardo DaVinci

120. Change the type of cardiovascular exercise you do every 4 – 6 weeks to keep your body changing. You won't get bored.

121. Cleaning the house? Put on some music and have fun dancing while cleaning.

122. Do something good while out in nature, bring a trash bag and gloves and pick up trash. Be a blessing to nature.

123. Toss the unhealthy snacks in the trash OR once you use them up, don't buy any more!

124. No time to do abdominal work? Ha! Pull your belly button in…let it out (repeat in a car, on a bus, airplane or checkout line at the market.)

125. Had to quit a workout early? Just do something extra a little later in the day….like taking a brisk walk.

126. Holiday season? Do your walking in the mall…you'll be shopping anyways and the bags will add weight to the workout.

"Tell me what you eat, and I shall tell you what you are."[xix]

Jean Anthelme Beillat-Savarin

127. Opt for natural butter instead of the chemical substitutes.

128. Rev up your calorie burning by Circuit Training: do one strength training exercise, then 1 minute of Cardio, move to the next strength exercise and repeat.

129. When riding a bike, don't get upset at catching a stop light or having to stop at a stop sign, use them for a type of speed work – see how quickly you can get back up to speed.

130. Allergies on a spring day? Use a bandana to block allergens or try Eucalyptus Oil or Ponaris to coat your nostrils.

131. Hot summer day? Do leg lifts and arm workouts in the pool using the water as resistance.

132. Got kids? Go play with them, play tag & really run!

133. Crave a specific food like cake from your local bakery? Wait 2 full days. Still craving? Go get one cupcake & thoroughly enjoy it. Now, go back to healthier choices. No guilt.

"A journey of a thousand miles must begin with a single step."[xx]

Lao Tzu

134. Going out for a celebration? Share the dessert!

135. Every time you finish a project (no matter how small,) celebrate by going for a short walk.

136. On the freeway? When you pass each major junction, correct your posture; sit up straight, tummy in. Head back.

137. If you have allergies, consider taking off your shoes at the front door so you don't track soil or pollen through the house.

138. Feeling drained after a hard workout? Replace your trace minerals (minerals your body needs in small amounts.)

139. Can't run…walk…can't walk, do chair aerobics.

140. Too stressed out to exercise? Go anyways, but imagine the person or issue causing the stress on the bottom of your shoes, on your palms or on the weights you are lifting… You can pound on them, slap them or just control that issue!

"Good health and good sense are two of life's greatest blessings."[xxi]

Publilius Syrus

141. Planning a decadent desert, eat fewer calories somewhere earlier in the day.

142. If you are planning a celebration, consider a cleanse or detox soon afterwards.

143. Oops, gained a pound or two? Just eat a little better today!

144. Write your fitness goals down. Read them aloud daily.

145. Read a book about someone who has overcome challenges on the way to becoming fit. It will inspire you!

146. Eat fruits at the beginning of your meal, it will help your digestion.

147. Want a 'perfect' body? Try to have YOUR best body, not some photo-shopped magazine image. Figure out what weight is the best for you and body fat % & go aim for that.

"The foundation of success in life is good health."[xxii]

P T Barnum

148. Take a rest day every now & then, but it can be active rest. Go take a walk with a friend.

149. If you want a quick and healthy lunch, blend 3 - 5 servings of fruit in a blender with some rice protein powder.

150. Find something healthy and interesting to try in your diet.

151. Get an accountability partner...hire a trainer to keep you accountable.

152. Evening snack? Try popcorn...it will fill you up on fewer calories.

153. Try cooking a meal with all healthy food: lots of veggies, pasta & fish.

154. Although it's great to have role models on your path to health, remember that they may have started from a different place. Start today & just work on improving a little bit at a time.

"May your light shine so brightly that those who have not yet found their light will be able to see their way through the dark."[xxiii]

Katrina Mayer

155. Give someone a hug…a 10-second hug will lower blood pressure by increasing Oxytocin and lowers the stress chemical, Cortisol.

156. Eating out? Try just drinking water. You can add lemon for flavor. No added calories.

157. A good nights sleep is restorative. If you have trouble getting to sleep, start a routine like writing down 5 things you are grateful for before bed, or reading 5 to 20 minutes.

158. If you go on a long walk with your dog, bring water for you & the dog. Make sure you BOTH drink.

159. Using an unfamiliar machine at a gym, have a staff member find someone to teach you how to properly use it or hire a trainer. Safety first!

160. Must study something? Try a stationary bike & read or study while exercising.

161. Take the stairs instead of the escalator or elevator.

"Faith is the substance of things hoped for, the evidence of things not seen."[xxiv]

Hebrews 11:1 (KJV)

162. Allow yourself one meal of your choice per week.

163. Don't want to sweat? At least get a "glow" on... Any release of moisture gets toxins out of your body!

164. Putting in extra hours at work & cannot workout? Eat a little less to avoid weight gain.

165. If you weigh yourself daily, you can keep track of progress or regress. Don't beat yourself up, but if you don't know the score, how will you know your progress?

166. Graph your weight progress so that you can nudge the number down or up to your goal.

167. Try, just for one day, not to eat ANY sugary sweets.

168. Feeling off? Like you may be getting a bug? Do a low intensity work out like an easy bike ride or walk & get some Vitamin D from the sun, if possible. And drink a lot of liquids.

"Our strength grows
out of our weakness."[xxv]

Ralph Waldo Emerson

169. After taking time off for illness or injury, start with shorter & easier work outs & build up to where you were.

170. Too hot outside? Go to a local ice skating rink, walk an indoor mall (avoiding the food court), swim or take an evening stroll.

171. If it's hot, consider alternating water & an electrolyte beverage.

172. Wear light colors when it's hot so they reflect the light & will keep you a little cooler.

173. Need a sweet desert with no added sugar. Try a pear or apple, cut in half, sprinkle with cinnamon and bake.

174. Having a scrumptious dinner? Choose healthier sides.

175. Holiday BBQ? Consider a burger wrapped in lettuce instead of a bun.

"Those who do not find time for exercise will have to find time for illness."[xxvi]

Edward Smith-Stanley

176. Craving chocolate or anything? Have a little bit & totally savor it.

177. When you travel by car, make sure to take a break every 2 hours & stretch your legs. You could even take a 5 minute walk around the rest stop or town where you stop.

178. Bring healthy snacks in the car so you aren't tempted by junk, or you can fill up on healthy snacks and get a small or kid's size meal.

179. If you plan a day in the sun, remember to put sunblock on top of your toes and on your ears.

180. Want to get faster in your sport? Do intervals of short fast bursts in between regular pace efforts.

181. Need to drink more water, but don't like plain water? Add a little lemon, lime juice, crushed mint or ginger.

182. Need sweetener? Try Stevia in the Raw instead of those chemical sweeteners.

"The groundwork of all happiness is health."[xxvii]

James Leigh Hunt

183. Hard work out & tired legs? Stretch.

184. If you have an upcoming race, do some speed work at the end of your long workouts so you are ready to push it on race day.

185. Need inspiration to exercise? Go volunteer at a hospital rehabilitation facility! When you see what they can do, you may be inspired to do more of what you can do.

186. If there's a chance of thunder, play indoors (dance around the house or plan a home strength program.)

187. Instead of juicing, try a smoothie. You will get all the nutrients & phyto-chemicals from the fruits & veggies.

188. Oops, ate too much last night? Today is a new day...eat a little less & a little healthier today!

189. Make sure the room you work out in is well ventilated with an air conditioner or fan.

"That which does
not kill me makes
me stronger."xxviii

Friedrich Nietzsche

190. When taking a walk, look at the scenery & smell the flowers.

191. Work on balance - stand on one leg for a minute. Then, the other...if that is too easy, try it standing on something narrow or unstable.

192. Get 7 - 8 hours sleep each night.

193. Didn't sleep well last night? Take a 20 minute power nap. Consider a guided meditation tape/audio.

194. Skip the appetizers & start with a salad. That starts the meal off healthy.

195. Kissing is good for the heart as well as the waistline. You can't eat & kiss at the same time!

196. If your stress levels are high, try deep breathing, meditation or yoga. It will calm you & lower your cortisol levels. High cortisol levels have shown to hold onto extra fat in the body.

"The beginning is the most important part of the work."xxix

Plato

197. If you feel stressed out about a situation, write out an affirmation for the day of the best possible outcome. Repeat it throughout the day.

198. Get regular medical check ups so that in case of an emergency, someone knows where your baseline (normal) is.

199. At work, always designate your preferred physician on your companies workman's compensation paper work so you can see them for issues that may arise.

200. Use a shopping trip as exercise: park in the furthest spot from the store & if you go to more than one store, put your bags in the car between stores (& don't walk slowly, hustle!)

201. Challenging diagnosis - get a second opinion - the treatment may be less stressful and you may learn different options.

202. If you want to wear flip flops, find some with arch support.

203. Waiting in line? Do calve raises or lunges for a quick workout.

"My great concern is not whether you have failed, but whether you are content in your failure."[xxx]

Abraham Lincoln

204. On a road trip? Bring a big cooler to keep beverages cool and healthy snacks in the car.

205. Hard workout or race? Consider an Epsom salts bath, menthol cream or a massage to facilitate healing.

206. Over indulged today? Stomach not feeling well? Try ginger or charcoal to calm it down.

207. If you're feeling down, have a music playlist or list of songs you can play that make you feel good. Play them to your favorite workout. Roller-skate??!!!?!?

208. If you don't want to carry water with you while you exercise, plan your route to go past water fountains or hoses.

209. Got a break? Stretch!

210. Stuck at a railroad crossing or traffic stop? Take the time to stretch, read a book or dance in your car. Keep the brake on.

"Nothing binds you except your thoughts; nothing limits you except your fear; and nothing controls you except your beliefs."[xxxi]

Marianne Williamson

211. If you must buy packaged food, keep the fat to less than 25% of total calories.

212. Eat less junk. Dance more.

213. Craving a specific food? Get a very small amount, but truly savor it. Take tiny bites & savor each one.

214. Waiting at the doctor's office? Work on your posture.

215. If you want to get faster in any sport, you have to do speed work. It trains the muscles how to get used to moving faster in short increments which will get faster the more you do it. Train fast, race fast...train slow, race slow.

216. If you have a hard time fitting in 60 minutes of exercise, try 20 minutes in the morning, 20 at lunch & 20 after work. It will keep you burning calories all day long.

217. If you feel nervous, fidget - it burns a few extra calories.

"It does not matter how slowly you go so long as you do not stop."xxxii

Confucius

218. Choose hair & body products with natural ingredients and no toxic chemicals. The skin takes in the toxins in your environment and what you put on your skin.

219. Want to be inspired to perspire? Volunteer at a charity athletic event. Seeing others do it will show you that you can, too!

220. Early for an appointment? Go for a short walk & burn off some extra calories.

221. Consider a 10 - 15 minute cold bath to cure your achey muscles (around 50 - 55 degrees Fahrenheit or 10 - 12.7 Celsius.)

222. Don't have time for a full workout? Half is better than nothing!

223. Bored with your diet? Try adding a new &/or exotic fruit or vegetable! Try kale, broccolini, sugar snap peas, papaya, or kiwi fruit.

224. Change the type of strength exercise you do every 4 - 6 weeks & your body will have to change to adapt. You will see greater changes in your body!

"No one knows what he can do until he tries."[xxxiii]

Publilius Syrus

225. Already dark outside? Use a flashlights, attachable lights or reflective clothing while you work-out outside.

226. If you are going out of town for a weekend, pack workout clothes. You'll at least be able to take a walk.

227. If it's really hot outside, shorten your workout or move it indoors.

228. Catching a late lunch? Stick to your meal plan & breathe in between bites.

229. Hotel gym full? Do stair repeats in your hotel, a nearby building or convention center.

230. Super sore from a new type of workout? Take it easy on those muscles with less weight/resistance.

231. If you feel you need a big purse or handbag, consider a backpack to fit over both shoulders or a rolling briefcase.

"Re-examine all that you have been told… dismiss that which insults your soul."xxxiv

Walt Whitman

232. Save Halloween candy in the freezer so you can enjoy one small candy per day instead of a big dessert.

233. Try green tea to replace at least one cup of coffee per day.

234. Already like dancing? Try a different type... Salsa, Swing, or Texas Two-step.

235. Use your computer or smart phone to find healthier restaurants in larger cities. In small towns, try to get food at local farmers markets.

236. If you are a caregiver for older parents, children or pets, be sure to take care of you with regular doctor visits, exercise, healthy food & massages!

237. Invest in a good pair of running shoes that fit and feel good. They are great, even for walking.

238. The choice is not skinny or happy...it's healthy or not! Easy choice!

"When the mind is pure, there is no fear."xxxv

Peter Ragnar

239. Do a detox or cleanse every 3 months/quarterly.

240. Don't FEEL like working out? Put on your workout clothes & imagine you when you hit your fitness goal. Get into that moment. How will you feel? Take at least 2 minutes to really feel the emotion. Now, go start your workout!

241. When you stretch, breathe into it and stretch for 30 seconds.

242. If it's very hot weather, consider waking up very early to exercise & taking a nap later.

243. In an area where there is snow? Go skiing! Downhill or cross-country.

244. Add some fiber to your salad or cereal - flax seeds, chia seeds or psyllium husk.

245. Get your regular medical, dental & vision checks...just to make sure everything is normal. Keep a copy of the results paperwork in your records.

"There is no struggle, there is no progress."[xxxvi]

Frederick Douglass

246. Find herbs or spices to flavor food instead of salt.

247. At that conference or meeting, consider bringing a bag or cooler with the food you choose to eat.

248. Need food, but don't know what you want? Try a smoothie with protein.

249. Spend some time breathing in some fresh air deep into your lungs. 5 - 10 minutes is optimal!

250. If you are doing a race, take the day before to rest your body. Walk from the parking lot to & around the expo as your only exercise for the day. (If it's a triathlon, consider driving the bike course & cycling the run course.)

251. While making copies at the office, march in place with high knees.

252. Read food labels & keep your fat intake below 25% on any item, and overall.

"To eat is a necessity, but to eat intelligently is an art."xxxvii

François de La Rochefoucauld

253. Walking to dinner? Put some music on the phone & walk to the beat!

254. Doing weights? Rest between sets to see better recovery & better results (& fewer injuries.)

255. If you have an active job, take time right after work to stretch.

256. Print or write your weight or health goal on a business card and refer to it while choosing from a menu. (Hold it in front of the menu.)

257. Bored of just walking? Put your earphones on with your favorite eras music & dance-walk!

258. Look for and eat LEAN meat or protein today.

259. If you have sore muscles from a new workout, get a massage. Go to a spa, a local massage school for their intern or your spouse, partner or friend.

"If you change the way you look at things, the things you look at change."[xxxviii]

Dr. Wayne Dyer

260. Rainy day? Play in the rain, choose appropriate gear.

261. Work your way up to 7 to 11 servings of fruits & veggies daily.

262. If you are attending a meeting or conference where there could be food that compromises your dietary goals, eat a very healthy meal before, so you can avoid too much junk.

263. Notice the things that you are doing right in your quest for abundant health. Make a list.

264. Feeling stressed? Do something, anything to feel better... Change your physiology: laugh, exercise, meditate, listen to your favorite song, hug a friend, smile!

265. Got somewhere early? Listen to some inspirational audio recordings!

266. If your legs are tired & sore from a workout after stretching, consider a 10-20min power nap with your legs up higher than your heart.

"A healthy body is a guest-chamber for the soul; a sick body is a prison."xxxix

Francis Bacon

267. Eat things that are God-made, not man-made 80-90% of the time or work your way there.

268. If you cannot pronounce an ingredient (unless you are a Science/Chemistry student,) don't eat or drink it!

269. Make a list on your computer of the things to avoid when shopping, listing food, vitamins, hair & body care items (i.e. high fructose corn syrup or magnesium stearate.) Carry the list with you when you shop.

270. When planning your exercise for the next day and packing a gym bag, remember toiletries, change of clothes, handi-wipes & all essentials you will need in a bag. In the morning you can just 'lock & load.'

271. Feeling sore? Consider arnica cream & stretching.

272. So you have to work a couple long days or attend a weekend seminar, consider a little extra work-out the day(s) before and after.

273. Tired? Try a B-vitamin complex.

"It takes courage… to endure the sharp pains of self discovery rather than the dull pain of unconsciousness that would last the rest of our lives."[xl]

Marianne Williamson

274. Ladies: if you are attending a party & must walk a ways to get there, bring some flats for walking & your heels for the party!

275. Watch for your favorite bands to come to town, go to the concert & dance the night away!

276. Feeling exhausted? Do a light workout or take an easy day. You may need a little extra rest.

277. See if your favorite restaurant has smaller portion sizes or share a meal.

278. If you know your schedule will become very busy soon, use a planner or calendar to schedule your exercise time. Try your smart phone calendar, google calendar or paper... but use it!

279. Freezer just died? What can you eat today? Donate the rest or toss it...DO NOT re-freeze!

280. Use exercise time as prayer or meditation time.

"Divide each difficulty into as many parts as is feasible and necessary to resolve it."[xli]

Rene Descartes

281. Ladies: are you having a neck or shoulder ache on one side? It could be your heavy purse. Either lighten the load or get a chic backpack.

282. Change from table salt (iodized) to sea salt.

283. If you know your schedule will be busy for a couple days with little or no workout time, cut back on your calories for those days.

284. Full at a family-style meal...either take a doggie bag or just say, "No, thanks!"

285. Legs sore from too much time in a car? Walk it off, stretch & use muscle easing cream.

286. If your muscles are cramping, you could be dehydrated. Drink an extra glass of water each day & more if you exercise more.

287. If you are feeling a little (or a lot) more stressed than usual, consider a longer workout to de-stress.

"Anything one man can imagine, other men can make real."[xlii]

Jules Verne

288. Want a decadent meal? Have a big salad & split the meal with a friend. You'll save calories & money!

289. Get your yearly physical & get a full blood panel. That will tell you if your diet is deficient in any nutrients.

290. Walking the dog & he constantly stops? Dance in place to keep your heart rate up!

291. Ladies… "That time of month?" Keep moving! Aside from keeping your fitness goals on schedule, it should lessen any PMS symptoms you may have. Men: help your partner keep moving.

292. If you will be flying, be sure to take your vitamins & maybe some extra vitamin C and D to protect against any germs.

293. Allergic to feathers or have special needs? Call ahead to your hotel & they will most likely accommodate your needs!

294. Eating out or at the airport? It's okay to leave food on your plate. Only eat until you feel slightly full.

"If you want to reach a goal, you must see the reaching in your own mind before you actually arrive at your goal."[xliii]

Zig Ziglar

295. Sightseeing? Pick a tour with some walking, hiking or cycling so you get your exercise in and see the beautiful sites.

296. Think you might go dancing? Bring comfortable shoes.

297. Learn to read labels to avoid harmful ingredients & chemicals in your food: consider carrying a printed list with you until you learn them.

298. If you are doing aerobic exercise, make sure you have carbohydrates in your system. Fruits or pasta are an option.

299. Weigh yourself every day. Not to cause worry, but to know exactly where you are with regards to your goal.

300. When on a cleanse, don't think 'What do I have to give up?' Think about 'What can I eat?' or 'What new and healthy things can I try?'

301. Goofed on the diet? Forgive yourself, move on & get back on it! One slip up won't hurt you.

"I saw few die of hunger; of eating, a hundred thousand."[xliv]

Benjamin Franklin

302. Really want to count calories? There's an app for that. Try the free ones first, then you can check out the pay ones.

303. Need to read (for school or work?) consider hopping on a stationary bike - regular or recumbent - put the bike on a program, then read & sweat! You can multitask! Hint: if you don't want to be bothered by talkers at the gym, put headphones in your ears. They don't have to know you have nothing playing.

304. Full from dinner? Take a walk or some light exercise, then, if needed, have a light dessert like baked pears with cinnamon.

305. Find a Farmer's Market near you & buy local foods.

306. Bring healthy snacks with you...some fruit & a handful of nuts are a great pick me up between meals.

307. Dance (turn on your stereo or headphones & boogie down.)

308. Instead of a cream sauce on meat or chicken, try a little extra virgin olive oil & some herbs.

"He who conquers
others is strong;
He who conquers
himself is mighty."[xlv]

Lao Tzu

309. If you want to live healthier, try food substitutions while cooking, like Olive oil for butter or Stevia for sugar.

310. If you are going to a potluck and you are on a restricted diet, bring something you want to eat that is healthy & filling.

311. If you bring your own lunch, you know you'll have something good to eat.

312. Having a challenge sticking to a healthier diet? Focus on your goal. Write it down on index cards & put them everywhere: on your mirror, refrigerator, door, office desk/computer, car visor. (Even better, get a picture of how you want to look.)

313. If you are thinking of your goal, focus on how you will feel when you reach it.

314. Add more veggies to your plate & less cheese.

315. If you try a new sport, you may have new muscle soreness, plan ice, bandaids or analgesic accordingly.

"The ancestor of every action is a thought."[xlvi]

Ralph Waldo Emerson

316. Eat protein with every meal or snack.

317. Take a good look at your body in the mirror (in the privacy of your own room) and focus at what is great about you.

318. Need a crunchy snack? Consider popcorn or better yet, carrots & sugar snap peas!

319. Bring your own healthy snacks to the movie theatre so you can control your calories & stay on track with your diet.

320. If your date cannot accommodate & support your dietary choices, don't accommodate him/her.

321. Don't like your doctor, try a new one with an attitude you like & who listens to you. Then you won't mind going.

322. If you don't have time to exercise or have to cut your workout short, just cut back on the portions you eat to balance out the calories.

"To preserve health is a moral and religious duty, for health is the basis of all social virtues. We can no longer be useful when we are not well."[xlvii]

Samuel Johnson

323. While exercising, tell yourself how great you'll feel when you are done.

324. Walk for 10 minutes on your lunch break.

325. If you have a slight injury (a body part you cannot use,) consider exercise that doesn't use that part. If it's your foot, swim or try pool running. If it's your hand or arm, try walking or stationary cycling. Maybe even just sit ups or crunches.

326. Read for 5 – 10 minutes before going to bed.

327. Nowadays, you can contact workout buddies & accountability partners by phone or texts. Use it to make workout plans.

328. Be proud of your workouts, post 'selfies' of you while you are working out on social media!

329. Floss your teeth, if not every day, then every other day. Harvard researchers have found a link between gum disease & heart attacks.

"Now's the day and now's the hour."[xlviii]

Robert Burns

330. Sleep better with the LED on your bedroom clock covered. Dim light at night has been shown to cause weight gain.

331. When you are on the phone, stand up & pace.

332. If you are waiting in line at a bank or store, you can do calve raises, squats or lunges. Maybe just take 4 deep 'belly' breaths.

333. Plan your workouts in your calendar (electronic or on paper,) it's important for you & the rest of your life to be healthy. Make you a priority!

334. Stretch after working out when the muscles are warm.

335. Want to try a new exercise and can not afford a trainer? Consider watching a video on how to do an exercise with a friend, then have that friend make sure you are doing it right!

336. Plan your food to fuel tomorrow's work-out, but don't try anything new on the day before an important race. You want to know how your body digests foods best! Bon appetit!

"Healing is a matter of time, but it is sometimes also a matter of opportunity."[xlix]

Hippocrates

337. When you finish a work-out, pat yourself on the back at your good job! You deserve it!

338. Skip the candlelight dinners. Studies show that bright light keeps you from eating as much.

339. Have some sweet flavored herbal tea around the house for an after dinner treat.

340. Instead of your standard pasta, try pasta made of rice (rice noodles) or Quinoa!

341. If you find a yummy, healthy dish a friend makes, ask them for the recipe. It's a compliment to the cook & then you can try it at home.

342. Chew Spry gum or another natural gum.

343. If you are coming up on a holiday that is centered around food, plan a good workout before the meal so you've burnt the calories before you eat them.

"The world cares about what we are. Our heart cares about who we are."

Aadil Palkhivala
"Fire of Love"

344. At a potluck or family dinner, consider a large salad & smaller portions of the main meal & sides.

345. Go to sleep 15 minutes earlier tonight.

346. Hungry? Or could it be thirst? Try a big glass of water first!

347. Do you have a 30 - 60 minute workout planned & don't feel like it? Just do 5 - 20 minutes, but see if you don't feel like doing the full workout once you get started.

348. If your body is used to exercising and you take a day off, remember to cut back on your caloric intake for the day.

349. Address your food issues and you've solved the biggest challenge with weight loss or gain. 80% of your body composition is a result of the food you put into it.

350. Instead of calling it 'eating food' consider changing that to 'fueling your body.'

"Health is a state of complete physical, mental and social well-being, and not merely the absence of disease or infirmity."[li]

Ralph Waldo Emerson

351. Break down your big goal into smaller mini-goals that are easier to attain.

352. Laugh at yourself. It will work the abs, too.

353. If you are doing an event, racing for competition or for fun, consider a very easy, light workout the day before the event.

354. Going out of town? Bring your own healthy food or do some internet research to find out where you can get healthy food at your destination and places in between, if it's a long journey.

355. In a town you don't know? Ask someone at the front desk for a healthy place to eat. If they don't know, stop by a local gym & ask.

356. Use the internet to find healthy, organic or vegan restaurants in your area or an area you are visiting. Try something new!

357. Find different herbs from different cultures to cook with. Try new things. If it's not that great, it was only one meal.

"If we could give every individual the right amount of nourishment and exercise, not too little and not too much, we would have found the safest way to health."[lii]

Hippocrates

358. Off to a party? If there's dancing, go for it! You can burn off some calories and have fun!

359. Don't need to go to the restroom during a break? Still, get up and take a short walk.

360. Drink filtered water without chemicals (Fluoride or Chlorine, etc.)

361. You can ask for food to be prepared more healthfully, like grilled chicken or a burger wrapped in lettuce instead of a bun.

362. If it's cold outside while you are working out, move faster... moving your muscles more increases the heat in your body.

363. Dress appropriately for the weather during your workout: if it's hot, wear light material of sweat dispersing material; if it's cold outside, wear warmer layers of moisture wicking material.

364. Waiting somewhere and cannot step away for a walk? Read something inspirational or listen to a positive audio. Or even write something for your book, a poem, or just a journal entry.

"It is not death that a man should fear, but he should fear never beginning to live."[liii]

Marcus Aurelius

365. Write down your fitness & health goals. Get pictures of them. Yes, even cut & paste your head on someone else's body. Then post the pictures on your Dream Board. Make sure your fitness goals are right in the middle!

366. (bonus for leap year) Meeting friends for coffee? Consider a low calorie, low fat option like non-fat latte or tea with Stevia. Skip the scones and opt for a piece of fruit.

End of one year...YOU DID IT!

Appendix A

List of different types of Fruit:

Apple
Apricot
Avocado
Banana
Breadfruit
Bilberry
Blackberry
Blackcurrant
Blueberry
Boysenberry
Cantaloupe
Currant
Cherry
Coconut
Cranberry
Cucumber
Date
Dragonfruit
Eggplant
Elderberry
Fig
Goji berry
Gooseberry
Grape (Raisin)
Grapefruit
Guava
Huckleberry
Honeydew

Jackfruit
Kiwi fruit
Kumquat
Lemon
Lime
Loquat
Lychee
Mango
Marion berry
Melon:
    Cantaloupe
    Honeydew
    Watermelon
Miracle fruit
Mulberry
Nectarine
Olive
Orange:
    Clementine
    Mandarine
    Blood Orange
    Tangerine
Papaya
Passionfruit
Peach
Pepper
    Chili pepper
    Bell pepper

Pear
Persimmon
Plum/prune (dried plum)
Pineapple
Pomegranate
Purple Mangosteen
Raspberry
Red Currant
Salmon berry
Satsuma
Star fruit
Strawberry
Tomato
Ugli fruit

Appendix B

List of Vegetables:

Artichoke

Arugula

Asparagus

Eggplant

Amaranth

Beens/Legumes:

    Alfalfa sprouts

    Azuki beans (or adzuki)

    Bean sprouts

    Black beans

    Black-eyed peas

    Broad beans

    Chickpeas, Garbanzos, or ceci beans

    Green beans

    Kidney beans

    Lentils

    Lima beans or Butter bean

    Mung beans

    Navy beans

    Pinto beans

    Soy beans

    Peas

    Snap peas

Beet

Bok choy

Broccoli

Brussels sprouts

Cabbage

Carrots

Cauliflower

Celery

Chard

Collard greens

Corn

Endive

Ginger

Herbs and spices

    Anise

    Basil

    Caraway

    Cilantro seed

    Chamomile

    Dill

    Fennel

    Lavender

    Lemon Grass

    Marjoram

    Oregano

    Parsley

    Rosemary

    Sage

    Thyme

Jicama
Kale
Lettuce
Mushrooms (actually a
fungus, not a plant)
Mustard greens
Nettles
Okra
Onion family
    Chives
    Garlic
    Leek
    Onion
    Shallot
Green onion/Scallion
Parsley
Parsnip
Peppers (actually fruits, but
treated as vegetables)
    Green pepper and Red
    pepper/ bell pepper/
    pimento
    Chili pepper/ Capsicum
    Jalapeno
    Habanero
    Paprika
    Tabasco pepper
    Cayenne pepper
Potato
Radicchio

Rhubarb
Rutabaga
Radish
    Horseradish
    Turnip
    Wasabi
    White radish
Spinach
Squashes (really fruits, but
treated as vegetables)
    Acorn squash
    Butternut squash
    Banana squash
    Zucchini (US)
    Cucumber (actually
    fruits, but treated as
    vegetables)
    Hubbard squash
    Squash
    Pumpkin
    Spaghetti squash
Sweet potato
Tomato (actually a fruit, but
treated as a vegetable)
Tubers
    Taro
    Yam
    Water chestnut
    Watercress

Appendix C

Chemicals to avoid

(in supplements, hair and body products.)

Shampoo & Conditioner:
Lauryl/Laureth Sulfates
Artificial scents
Dyes
Preservative
Animal based ingredients
Facial Cleansers:
Petroleum based
Artificial Preservatives
Sodium Lauryl/Laureth
Sulphate
Parabens (methyl-, ethyl-, and butyl-)
Synthetic colors/scents
Unpurified Water with
Chlorine
Facial Moisturizers:
Petroleum based
Artificial Ingredients
Parabens (methyl-, ethyl-, and butyl-)
Synthetic colors
Synthetic scents
Animal based ingredients
Supplements:
Magnesium Stearate
Stearic Acid
Talc
All Products:

Alkyloamides:
DEA - diethanolamides
MEA - monoethanolamides
TEA - triethanolamides
MIPA - momoisopropanolamides
PEG - ethoxylated alkyloamides
Aluminum
Alcohol
Aminomethyl Propanol
Broax
BHT - Butylated Hydroxianisole
BHA - Butylated Hydroxytoluene
FD&C - Blue Dye 1, Green 3, Red 33, Yellow 5 & 6
Disodium EDTA
Ethylene/Acrylic Acid Copolymer
Phthalates
Glycerol Oleate
Oxybenzone
Sodium Hydroxide
Triethanolamine
Talc
Silicone derived emollients

Appendix D

Statistics

Height _____

Age _____

Starting	Mid-Year	End of Year
Body Fat % _____	Body Fat % _____	Body Fat % _____
Weight _____	Weight _____	Weight _____
Resting HR _____	Resting HR _____	Resting HR _____
Neck _____	Neck _____	Neck _____
Chest _____	Chest _____	Chest _____
Bicep R/L ____/_____	Bicep R/L ____/_____	Bicep R/L ____/_____
Forearm R/L ___/____	Forearm R/L ____/____	Forearm R/L ____/____
Waist _____	Waist _____	Waist _____
Hips _____	Hips _____	Hips _____
Thigh R/L _____/____	Thigh R/L _____/____	Thigh R/L _____/____
Calf R/L _____/_____	Calf R/L _____/_____	Calf R/L _____/_____
BMI _____	BMI _____	BMI _____

End Notes

i   Ralph Waldo Emerson, "Society and Solitude" (1870)

ii   Abraham Lincoln (Letter to Isham Reavis 11-5-1855)

iii   Vincent Van Gogh (Letter to Theo, October 1882)

iv   Ed Foreman - U.S. Congressman (Ret.) Texas & New Mexico, Author, Speaker, Entrepreneur; spoken to Global Information Network event 2014.

v   Marcus Valerius Martialis (Epigrams c.80-104AD, VI, 70.)

vi   Marcus Aurelius (121 A D - 180A D) https://www.goodreads.com/quotes/64212-the-happiness-of-your-life-depends-upon-the-quality-of

vii   Henri Frederic Amiel (1828 - 1881) https://www.brainyquote.com/quotes/h/henrifrede383445.html

viii   Theodore Roosevelt (written in Charlotte (NC) Observer 7/14/1895.)

ix   Johann Wolfgang von Goethe (1749 -1832) https://www.brainyquote.com/quotes/quotes/j/johannwolf161315.html

x   Thomas Huxley (1825 - 1895) https://www.brainyquote.com/quotes/t/thomashuxl101466.html

xi   Jessica Ortner "Tapping for Weight Loss" 2014

xii   Aristotle (384 BC - 322 BC) https://www.brainyquote.com/quotes/quotes/a/aristotle145967.html

xiii   Buddha *(563 BC - 483 BC)* https://www.brainyquote.com/quotes/b/buddha387356.html

xiv   Elbert Hubbard (Electrical Review c. 1895)

xv   1 Corinthians 3:16 (KJV)

xvi   Thomas Carlyle (1795 - 1881) https://www.brainyquote.com/quotes/t/thomascarl118220.html

xvii   Confucius (551 BC - 479 BC) https://www.brainyquote.com/quotes/c/confucius101164.html

xviii   Leonardo DaVinci (1452 -1519) https://www.goodreads.com/quotes/8684-one-can-have-no-smaller-or-greater-mastery-than-mastery

xix   Jean Anthelme Beillat-Savarin Physiologie du Gout (1825)

xx   Lao Tzu (Tao Te Ching)

xxi   Publilius Syrus (1st Century BC) https://www.brainyquote.com/quotes/quotes/p/publiliuss391791.html

xxii   P T Barnum (1810 -1891) https://www.brainyquote.com/quotes/quotes/p/ptbarnum539969.html

xxiii   Katrina Mayer www.katrinaswholarianvision.com Wholarian Vision, 2011

xxiv   Hebrews 11:1 (KJV)

xxv   Ralph Waldo Emerson "Essays: First Series (Compensation)" 1841

xxvi   Edward Smith-Stanley (14th Earl of Derby, 1752 - 1834) http://www.searchquotes.com/quotation/Those who do not find time for exercise will have to find time for illness./301725/

xxvii   James Leigh Hunt *(1784-1859)* http://izquotes.com/quote/89622

xxviii   Friedrich Nietzsche (Twilight of the Idols, 1888)

xxix   Plato (The Republic, Book II, ~380AD)

xxx   Abraham Lincoln (16th President of the United States of America 1809 - 1865) http://thinkexist.com/quotation/my great concern is not whether you have failed/12575.html

xxxi   Marianne Williamson "The Law of Divine Compensation" Harper Collins 2014

xxxii   Confucius (551 BC – 479 BC) http://www.quotationspage.com/quote/3132.html

xxxiii   Publilius Syrus (Sentances, Maxim 786)

xxxiv   Walt Whitman (1819 -1892) https://www.brainyquote.com/quotes/quotes/w/waltwhitma130659.html

xxxv   Peter Ragnar www.longevitysage.com

xxxvi   *Frederick Douglass (Address on West India Emancipation 8-3-1857)*

xxxvii   *François de La Rochefoucauld (1613 - 1680) To eat is a necessity, but to eat intelligently is an art.*

xxxviii   Dr. Wayne Dyer http://www.inspirationalquotes4u.com/dyerquotes/index.html

xxxix   Francis Bacon *(1561 -1626)* http://www.searchquotes.com/quotes/author/Francis Bacon/

xl   Marianne Williamson "A Return to Love: Reflections on the Principles of "A Course in Miracles" Harper Collins 1996

xli   Rene Descartes "Le Discours de la Méthode", 1637

xlii   Jules Verne "Around the World in Eighty Days" 1873.

xliii   Zig Ziglar 1926 - 2012) http://www.ziglar.com/quotes/if-you-want-reach-goal

xliv   *Benjamin Franklin (1706 - 1790)* http://www.quotedb.com/quotes/1003

xlv   Lao Tzu "Tao Te Ching"

xlvi   Ralph Waldo Emerson "Essays: First Series" Spiritual Laws, 1841

xlvii	Samuel Johnson (English Poet, Critic and Writer, 1809 www.finestquotes.com/select_quote-category-Health-page
xlviii	Robert Burns "Scots Wha Hae",(1794)
xlix	Hippocrates (460 BC - 377 BC) http://www.quotationspa, quote/24180.html
l	Aadil Palkhivala "Fire of Love" 2008
li	Ralph Waldo Emerson (1803 - 1882) http://thinkexist.com/quotatio, health_is_a_state_of_complete_physical-mental_and/188294.html
lii	Hippocrates (460 BC - 377 BC) https://www.brainyquote.com/quotes/ quotes/h/hippocrate153531.html
liii	Marcus Aurelius (121 AD - 180 AD)https://www.brainyquote.com/ quotes/quotes/m/marcusaure148732.html

Made in the USA
San Bernardino, CA
25 July 2016